What's In It For Me?

By Wyatt Michaels

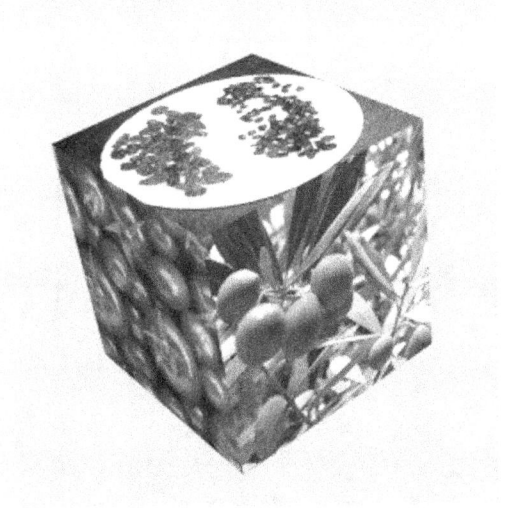

Images courtesy of meaduva (olives), Joanna Bourne (raisins), and The Ewan (tomatoes)

Which of these are fruit?

A. Olives
B. Raisins
C. Tomatoes
D. All the above.

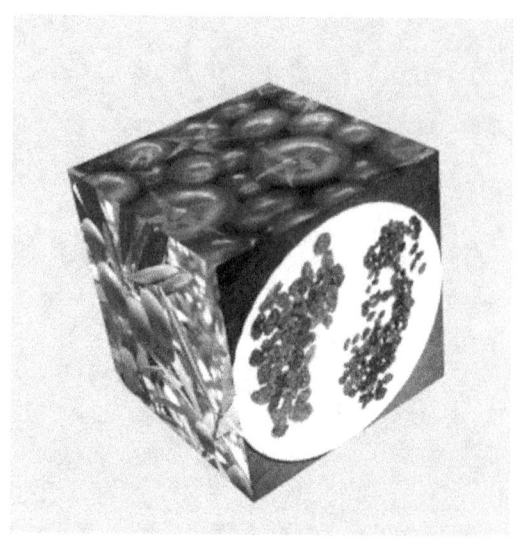

Images courtesy of meaduve, Joanna
Bourne, and the Ewan

The answer is D. All the above

Olives, raisins (dried grapes) and
tomatoes are all considered to
be fruit.

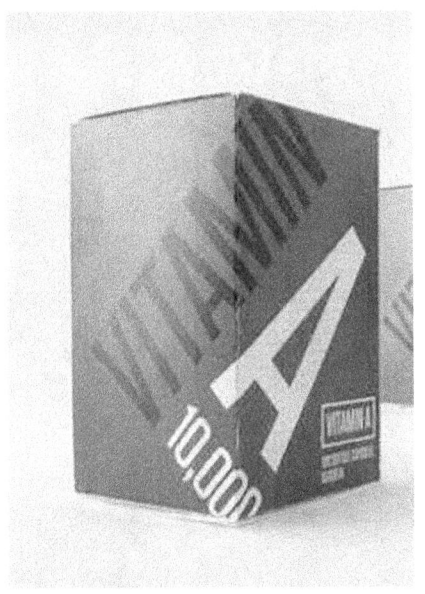

Image courtesy of colindunn

Which fruit provides more than 100% of recommended daily intake of Vitamin A?

A. Cantaloupe
B. Lemons
C. Mango

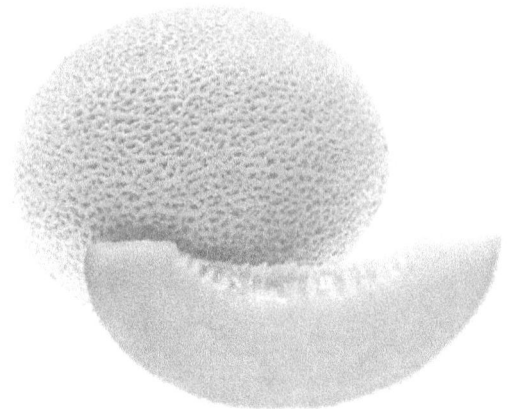

Image courtesy of public domain

The answer is A. Cantaloupe

One medium wedge of cantaloupe provides approximately 116% of the recommended daily intake of vitamin A. One lemon (without the peel) provides less than 1% of the recommended daily intake of vitamin A. One mango (without the peel) provides almost 80% of the recommended daily intake of vitamin A.

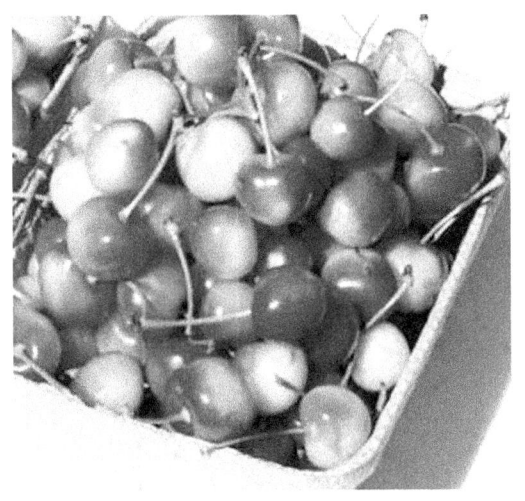

Image courtesy of La Grande Farmers' Market

Cherries contain the highest percentage of which vitamin?

A. Vitamin B1
B. Vitamin C
C. Folate

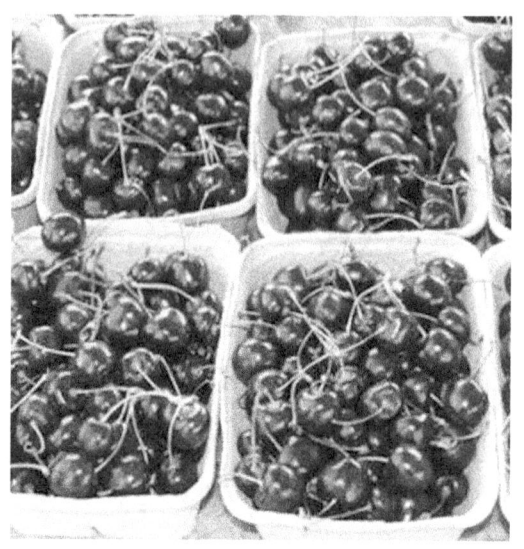

Image courtesy of La Grande Farmers' Market

The answer is B. Vitamin C

One cup of cherries provides over 12% of the recommended daily intake of vitamin C. It provides less than 3% of the recommended daily intake of vitamin B1 and less than 2% of the recommended daily intake of Folate (a B vitamin).

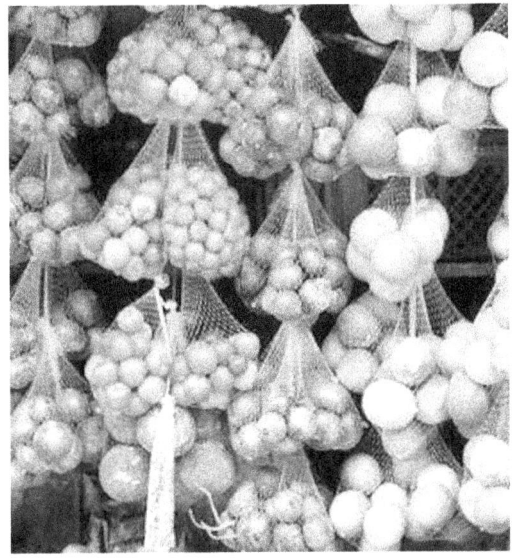

Image courtesy of Jonny D Green

Which fruit provides the most protein?

    A. Cantaloupe

    B. Pears

    C. Pomegranates

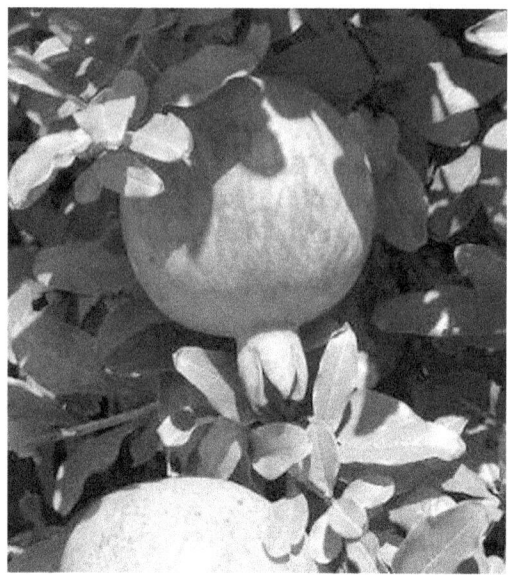

Image courtesy of garlandcannon

The answer is C. Pomegranates

One pomegranate provides almost 5 grams of protein. One medium wedge of cantaloupe provides less than 1 gram of protein. One medium pear provides less than 1 gram of protein.

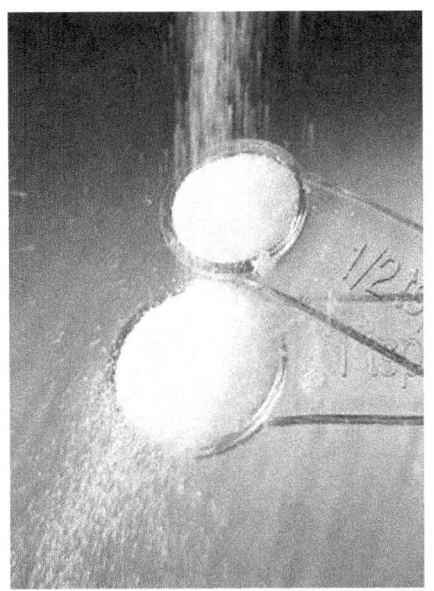

Image courtesy of USDA

Which fruit has minimal vitamin and mineral value except for sodium?

A. Avocado
B. Beets
C. Olives

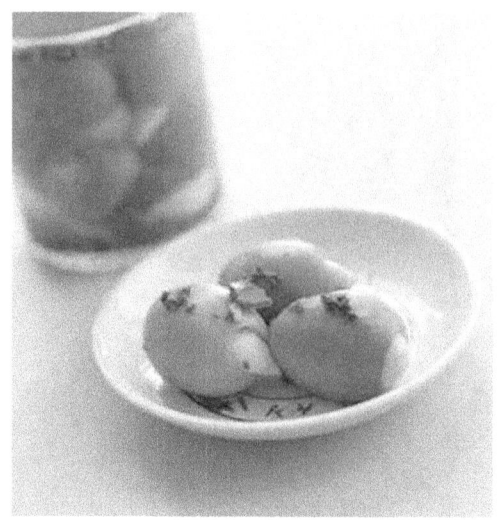

Image courtesy of ninacoco

The answer is C. Olives

The nutritional value of olives comes from their anti-oxidant and anti-inflammatory and other benefits and not strictly from common vitamins and minerals. Avocados are full of vitamins and minerals. Beets have sodium, but they are a root and not a fruit.

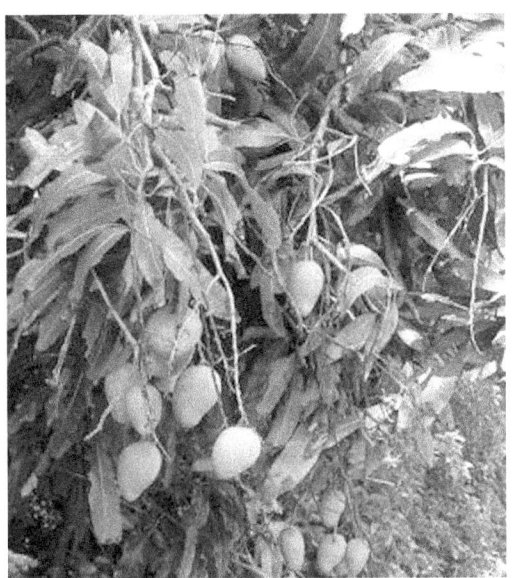

Image courtesy of 4nitsirk

Mangos contain the highest percentage of which vitamin?

A. Vitamin A
B. Vitamin B1
C. Vitamin B2

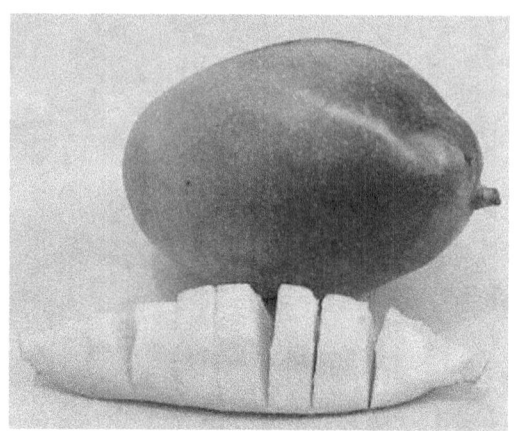

Image courtesy of richard north

The answer is A. Vitamin A

One mango (without peel) provides almost 80% of the recommended daily intake of vitamin A. It provides less than 9% of the recommended daily intake of vitamin B1 and less than 8% of the recommended daily intake of vitamin B2.

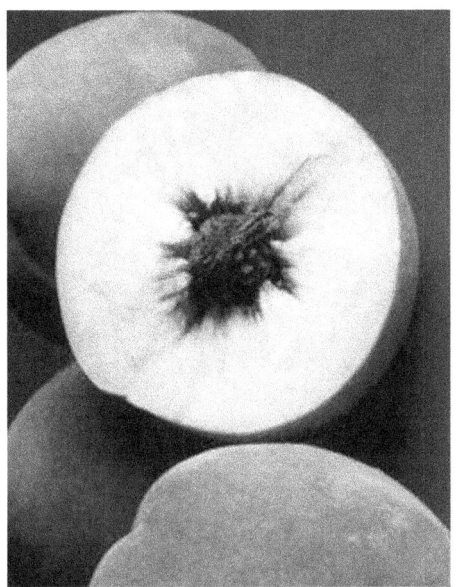

Image courtesy of public domain

Peaches contain the highest percentage of which vitamin?

A. Niacin
B. Vitamin A
C. Vitamin B1

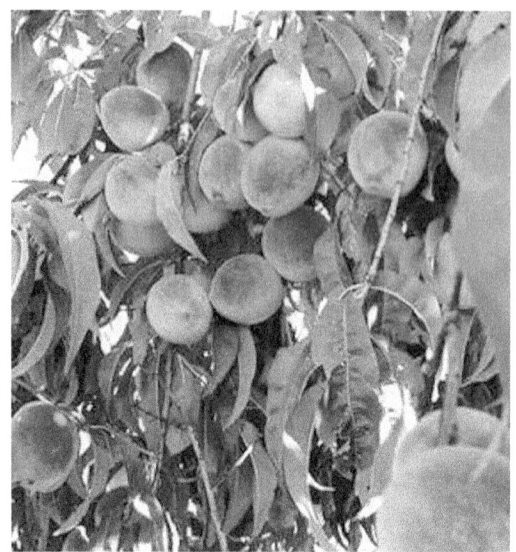

Image courtesy of sociotard

The answer is B. Vitamin A

One medium peach provides almost 25% of the recommended daily intake of vitamin A. It provides less than 7% of the recommended daily intake of niacin and less than 3% of the recommended daily intake of vitamin B1.

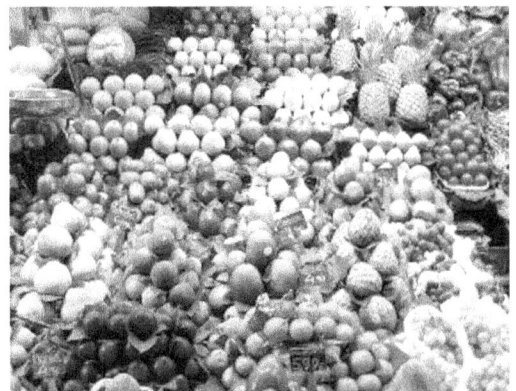

Image courtesy of theseanster93

If you wanted the most of the mineral potassium possible, which fruit should you eat?

    A. Avocado
    B. Banana
    C. Pomegranate

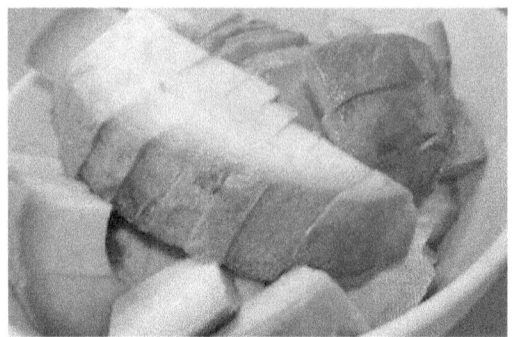

Image courtesy of Andreanna Moya
Photography

The answer is A. Avocado

One medium avocado provides almost 28% of the recommended daily intake of potassium. Bananas are known for providing potassium, and they do a good job of supplying over 12% of the recommended daily intake. Pomegranates provide over 19% of the recommended daily intake of potassium.

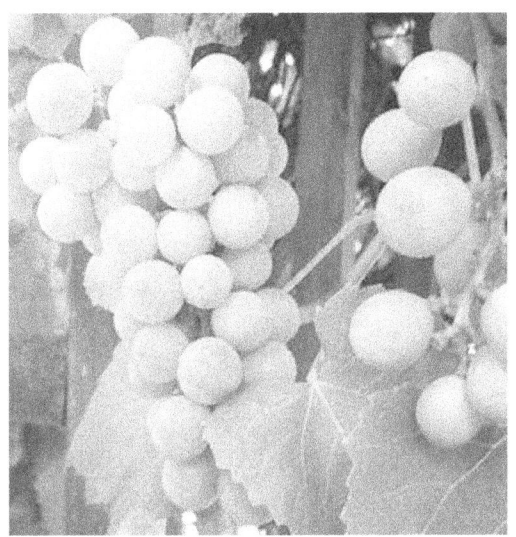

Image courtesy of Jeena Paradies

Grapes contain the highest percentage of which vitamin?

A. Vitamin B2
B. Vitamin B6
C. Vitamin K

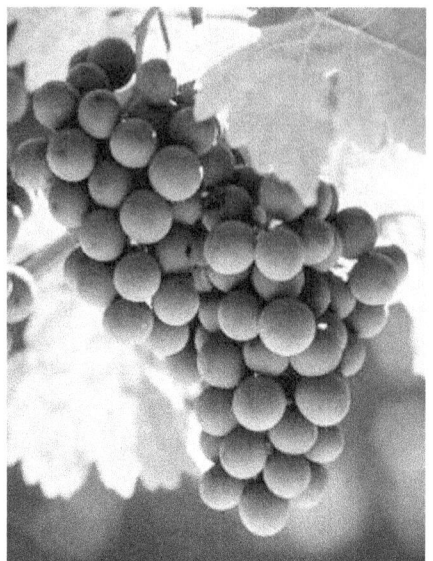

Image courtesy of Zest-pk

The answer is C. Vitamin K

One cup of grapes provides over 27% of the recommended daily intake of vitamin K. They provide just less than 7% of vitamin B2 and 6-7% of the recommended daily intake of vitamin B6.

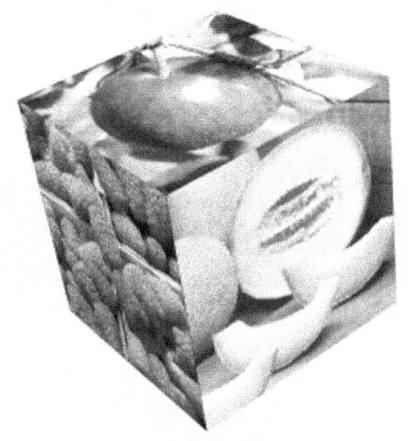

Images courtesy of public domain
(apples, cantaloupe) and La Grande
Farmers' Market (raspberries)

Of these three fruits, which one
has the highest percentage of
Vitamin C?

    A. Apples
    B. Cantaloupe
    C. Raspberries

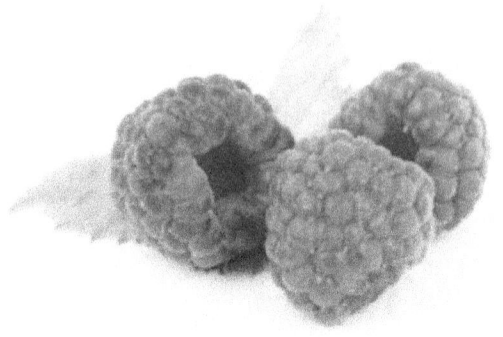

Image courtesy of public domain

The answer is C. Raspberries

One cup of raspberries provides about 42% of the recommended daily intake of vitamin C. One medium apple provides about 11% and one medium wedge of cantaloupe provides about 34% of the recommended daily intake of vitamin C.

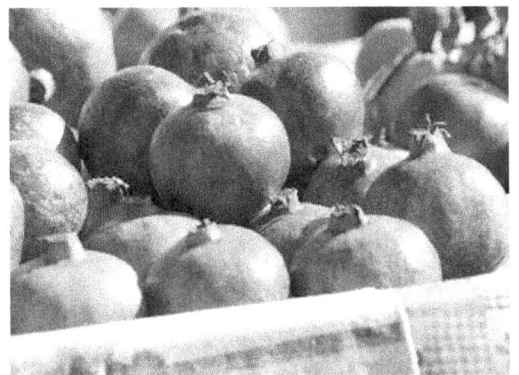
Image courtesy of John-Morgan

Pomegranates contain the highest percentage of which vitamin?

A. Vitamin B1
B. Vitamin E
C. Vitamin K

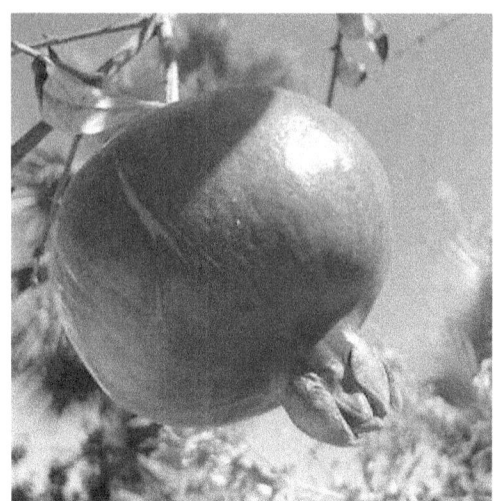

Image courtesy of Mari Smith

The answer is C. Vitamin K

Pomegranates have a high percentage of many vitamins, but they are highest in vitamin K with about 58% of the recommended daily intake. One fresh pomegranate provides over 13% of the recommended daily intake of vitamin B1 and almost 17% of the recommended daily intake of vitamin E.

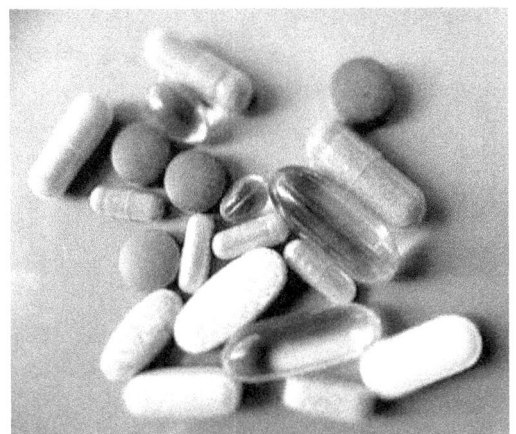

Image courtesy of shannonkringen

Which fruit provides the most recommended daily Vitamin B2?

A. Avocado
B. Bananas
C. Tomatoes

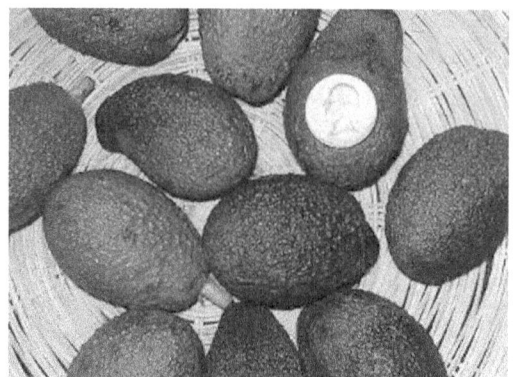

Image courtesy of miheco

The answer is A. Avocado

Avocados are very high for many vitamins, and they are the highest in this category, with one medium avocado providing over 16% of the recommended daily intake of vitamin B2. One medium banana provides over 5% and one medium tomato provides less than 2% of the recommended daily intake.

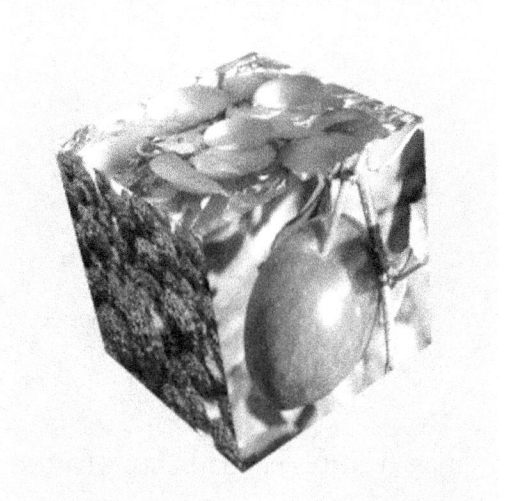

Images courtesy of public domain (apple), Different Seasons Jewelry (boysenberries) and Neville10 (grapefruit)

Of these three fruits, which one has the highest percentage of selenium?

A. Apple
B. Boysenberries
C. Grapefruit

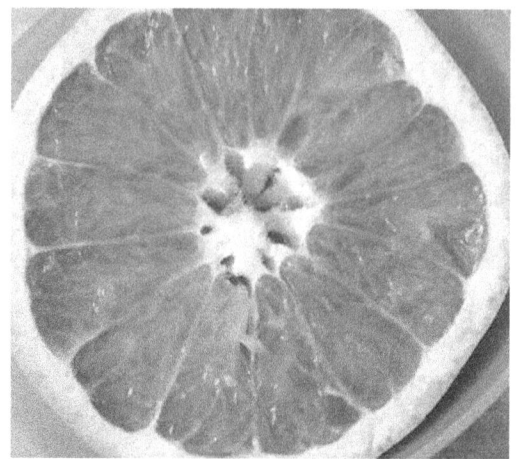

Image courtesy of Barbara L. Hanson

The answer is C. Grapefruit

One cup of grapefruit provides about 2% of the trace element, selenium. Apples provide little to no selenium. And one cup of frozen boysenberries provides about 1% of the recommended daily intake of selenium.

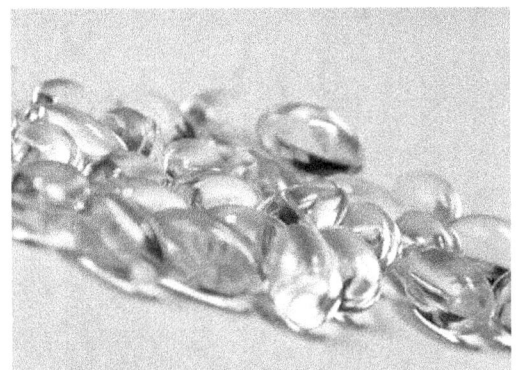

Image courtesy of LifeSupercharger

If you wanted the most Vitamin E possible, which one of these three fruits should you eat?

A. Cherries
B. Mango
C. Peaches

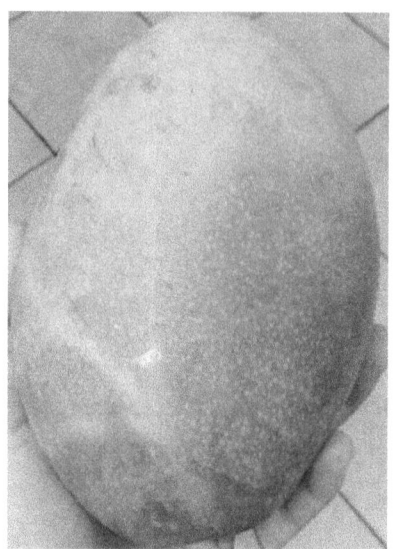

Image courtesy of Zenia Nunez

The answer is B. Mango

One mango (without peel) provides about 23% of the recommended daily intake of vitamin E. Only an avocado has more. One cup of cherries only provides about 1% and one medium peach provides almost 11% of the recommended daily intake of vitamin E.

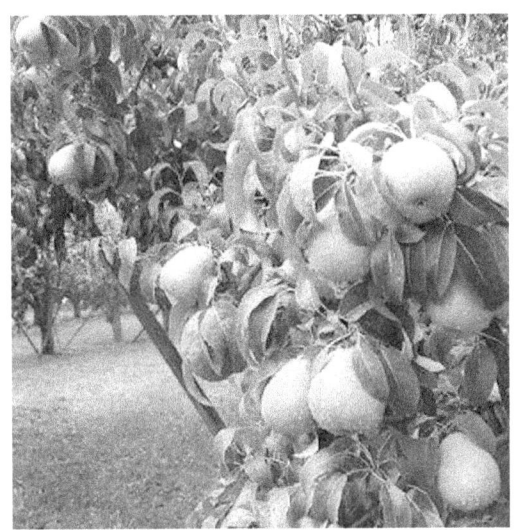

Image courtesy of pjsixft

Pears contain the highest percentage of which vitamin?

   A. Vitamin B2
   B. Vitamin K
   C. Folate

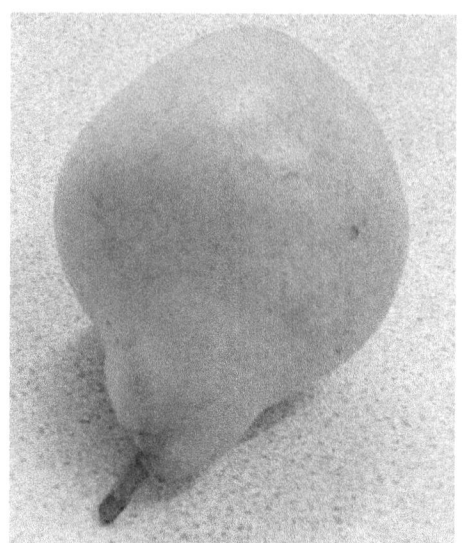

Image courtesy of richard north

The answer is B. Vitamin K

One medium pear provides about 10% of the recommended daily intake of vitamin K (as well as vitamin C). One medium pear provides almost 3% of the recommended daily intake of vitamin B2 and 3% of the recommended daily intake of Folate.

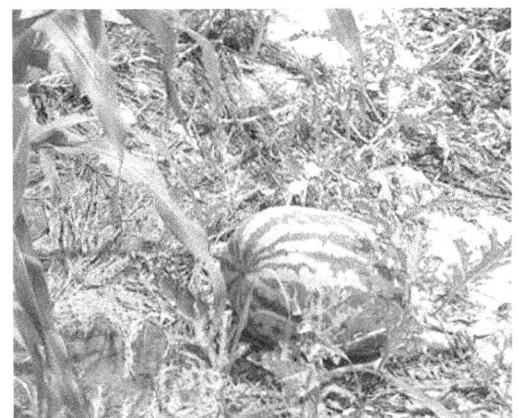

Image courtesy of Jason Riedy

Watermelon contains the highest percentage of which vitamin?

A. Vitamin A
B. Vitamin B2
C. Vitamin C

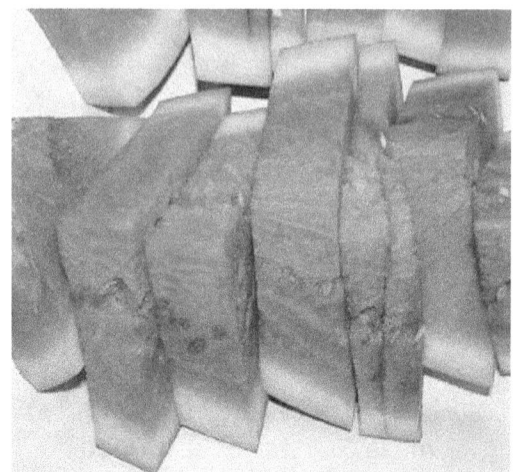

Image courtesy of lcstravelbuggin

The answer is A. Vitamin A

Two cups of watermelon provide about 81% of the recommended daily intake of vitamin A. It provides less than 4% of the recommended daily intake of vitamin B2 and about 30% of the recommended daily intake of vitamin C.

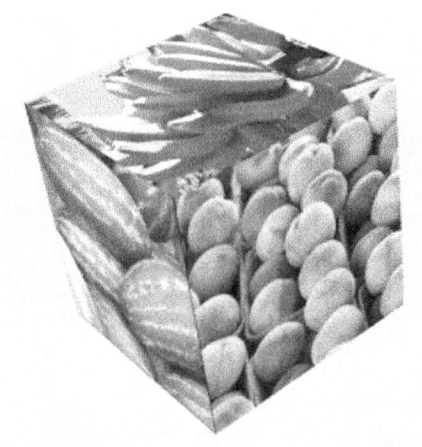

Images courtesy of librarianidol
(bananas), and La Grande Farmers
Market (peaches and watermelon)

Of these three fruits, which one
has the highest percentage of
Pantothenic Acid?

A. Bananas
B. Peaches
C. Watermelon

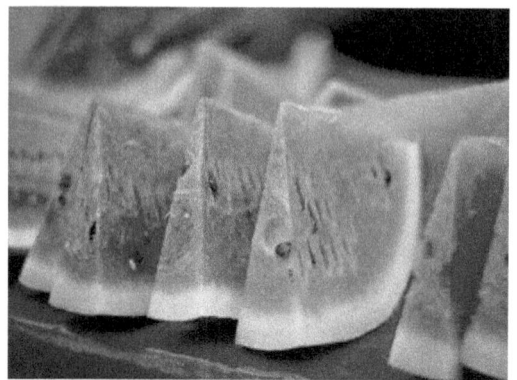

Image courtesy of mynameisharsha

The answer is C. Watermelon

Two cups of watermelon provides over 10% of the recommended daily intake of Pantothenic Acid. Avocados and pomegranates provide even more than that. One medium banana provides over 6% and one medium peach provides less than 4% of the recommended daily intake of pantothenic acid.

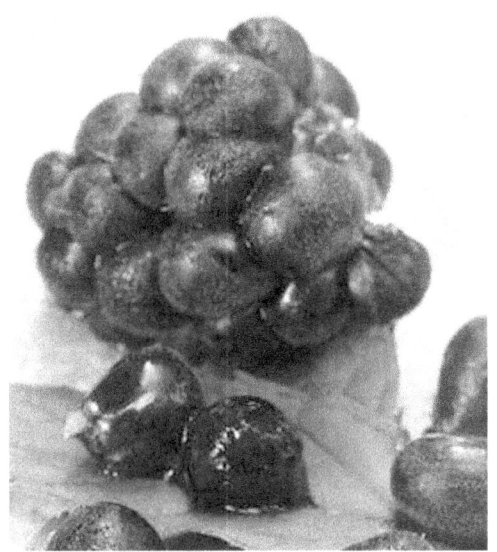

Image courtesy of Eran Finkle

Boysenberries contain the highest percentage of which vitamin?

A. Vitamin B6
B. Folate
C. Niacin

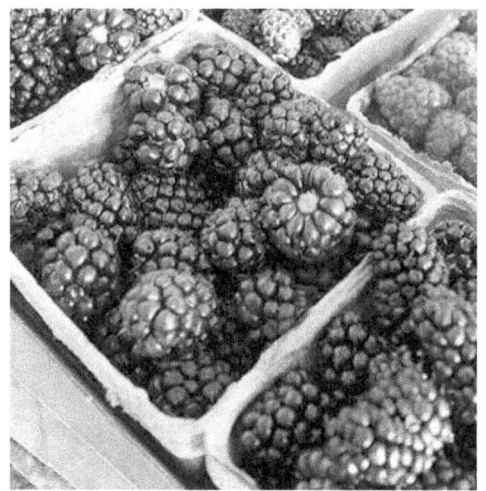

Image courtesy of Jon Rohan

The answer is B. Folate

Two cups of frozen boysenberries provide over 20% of the recommended daily intake of Folate. Only avocados and pomegranates provide more. One cup of frozen boysenberries provides less than 4% of the recommended daily intake of vitamin B6 and just less than 6% of the recommended daily intake of niacin.

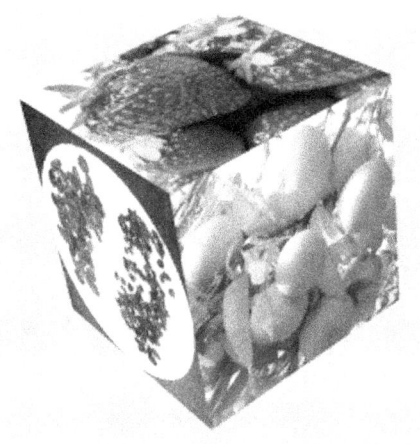

Images courtesy of Neville10
(grapefruit), Joanna Bourne (raisins),
and seelensturm (strawberries)

Of these three fruits, which one
has the highest percentage of
phosphorus?

    A. Grapefruit
    B. Raisins
    C. Strawberries

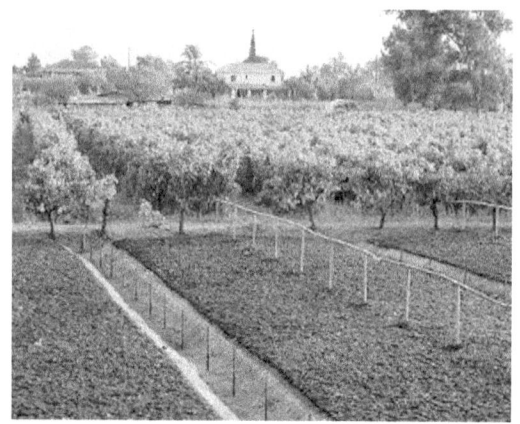

Image courtesy of RobW

The answer is B. Raisins

One small box of raisins provides more than 4% of the recommended daily intake of phosphorus. One cup of grapefruit provides less than 2% and one cup of whole strawberries provides about 3.5% of the recommended daily intake of phosphorus.

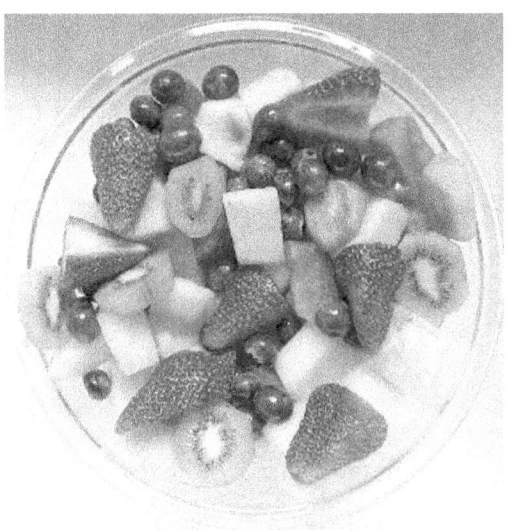

Image courtesy of lisaclarke

Which fruit gives you the highest percentage of Vitamin B6?

A. Cantaloupe
B. Grapefruit
C. Strawberries

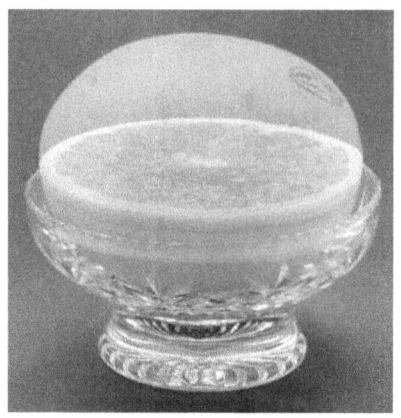

Image courtesy of exfordy

The answer is B. Grapefruit

One cup of grapefruit provides almost 5% of the recommended daily intake of vitamin B6. Other fruits such as avocado, bananas, mangos, and pomegranates provide 10 to 25% of the recommended daily intake. One medium wedge of cantaloupe provides less than 3% and one cup of whole strawberries provides just over 3% of the recommended daily intake of vitamin B6.

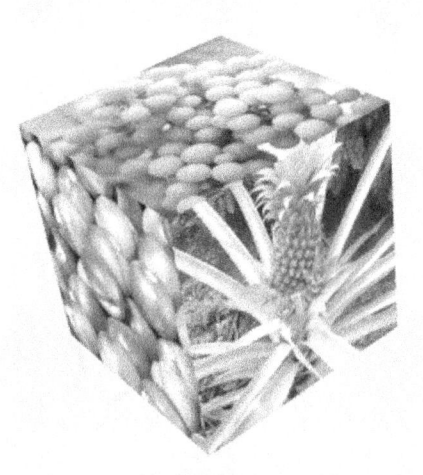

Images courtesy of tribp (grapes),
TheGirlsNY (nectarines), and
derek7272 (pineapple)

Of these three fruits, which one
has the highest percentage of
magnesium?

A. Grapes
B. Nectarines
C. Pineapple

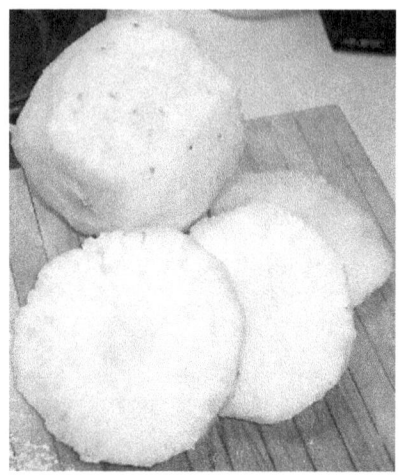

Image courtesy of the bridge

The answer is C. Pineapple

One cup of fresh pineapple chunks provides almost 6% of the recommended daily intake of magnesium. Avocados, blackberries, bananas, watermelon and pomegranates provide more than 6%. One cup of grapes provides just over 3% and one cup of sliced nectarines provides just less than 4% of the recommended daily intake of magnesium.

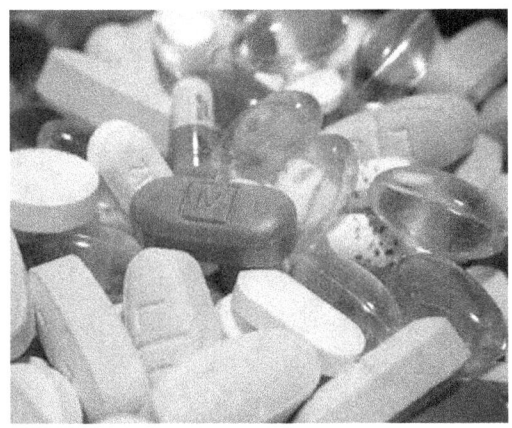

Image courtesy of stevendepolo

Which fruit gives you the highest percentage of most vitamins and minerals?

    A. Avocado
    B. Cantaloupe
    C. Cherries

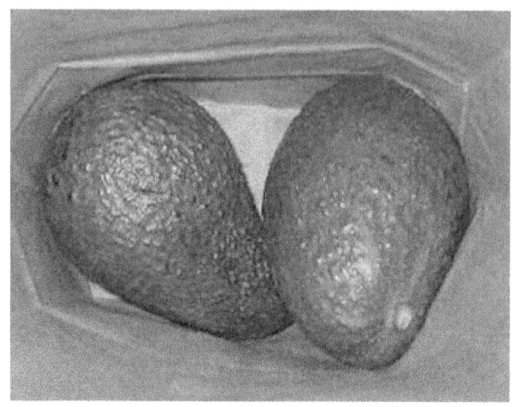

Image courtesy of nate steiner

The answer is A. Avocado

One medium avocado provides a high percentage vitamin A, B1, B2, niacin, Folate, pantothenic acid, B6, C, E, and K as well as the minerals potassium, phosphorus, magnesium, sodium, iron, and copper.

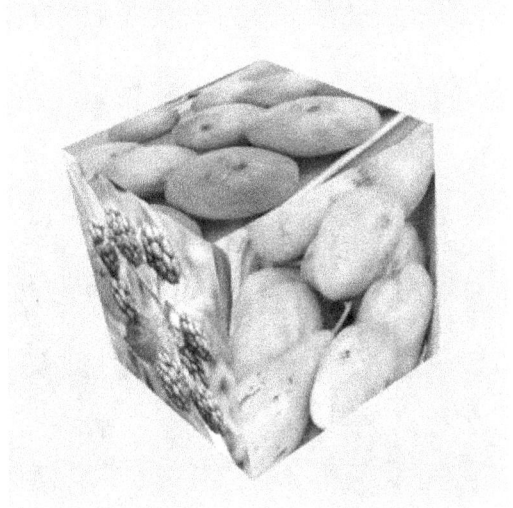

Images courtesy of public domain (blackberries), FutureExpat (mango), and La Grande Farmers Market (pears)

Of these three fruits, which one has the highest percentage of Vitamin K?

   A. Blackberries
   B. Mango
   C. Pears

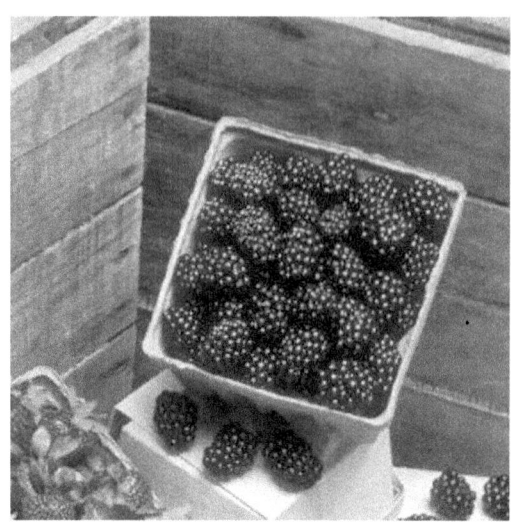

Image courtesy of public domain

The answer is A. Blackberries

One cup of blackberries proved over 35% of the recommended daily intake of vitamin K. One mango (without peel) provides almost 11% and one medium pear provides about 10% of the recommended daily intake of Vitamin K.

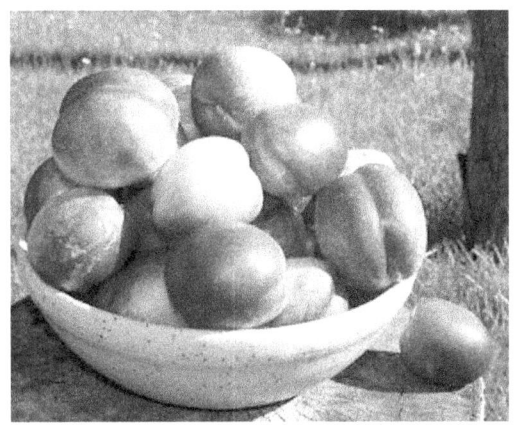

Image courtesy of sand and sky

Nectarines contain the highest percentage of which vitamin?

- A. Folate
- B. Vitamin A
- C. Vitamin B6

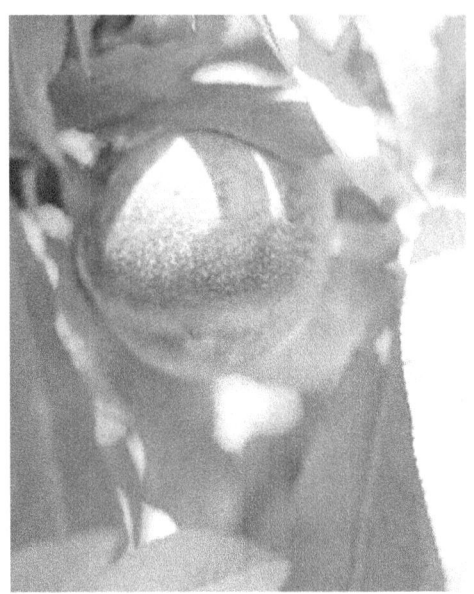

Image courtesy of Living in Monrovia

The answer is B. Vitamin A

One cup of sliced nectarines provides almost 24% of the recommended daily intake of vitamin A. It provides less than 2% of the recommended daily intake of Folate and less than 2% of the recommended daily intake of vitamin B6.

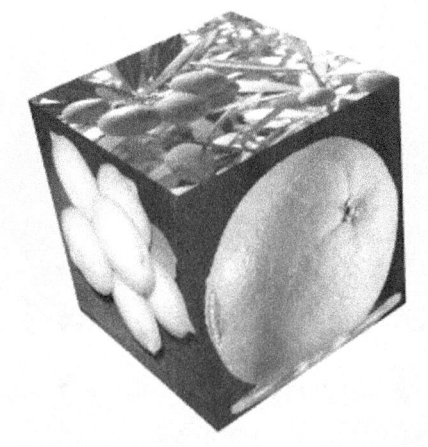

Images courtesy of Golf Bravo1 (lemons), meaduva (olives), and The Ewan (orange)

Of these three fruits, which one has the highest percentage of calcium?

    A. Lemons
    B. Olives
    C. Oranges

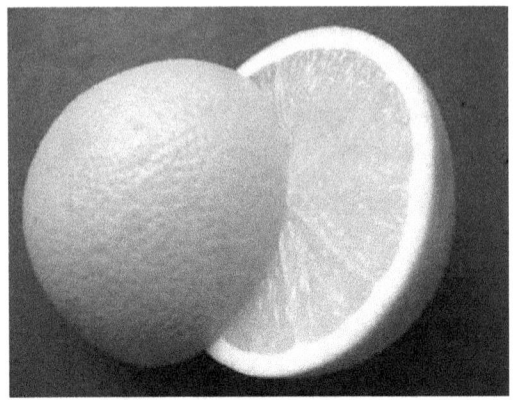

Image courtesy of public domain photos

The answer is C. Oranges

One medium orange provides more than 5% of the recommended daily intake of calcium. One lemon (without peel) provides less than 3% and one tablespoon of olives provides less than 1% of the recommended daily intake of calcium.

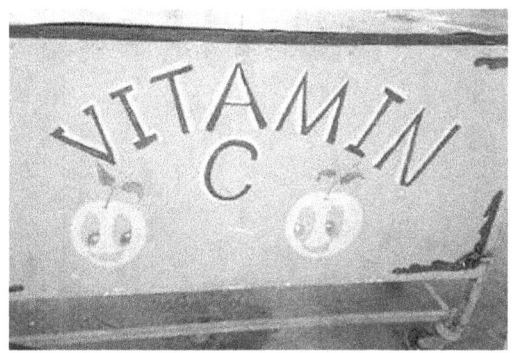

Image courtesy of JMR Photography

Which fruit provides more than 100% of recommended daily intake of Vitamin C?

A. Blackberries
B. Oranges
C. Strawberries

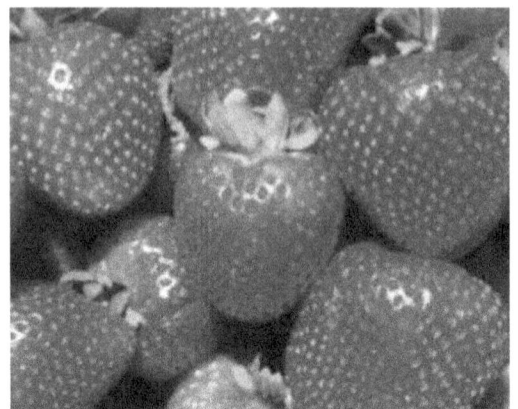

Image courtesy of public domain

The answer is C. Strawberries

One cup of whole strawberries provides about 113% of the recommended daily intake of vitamin C. One cup of blackberries provides about 40% and one medium orange "only" provides about 93% of the recommended daily intake of vitamin C.

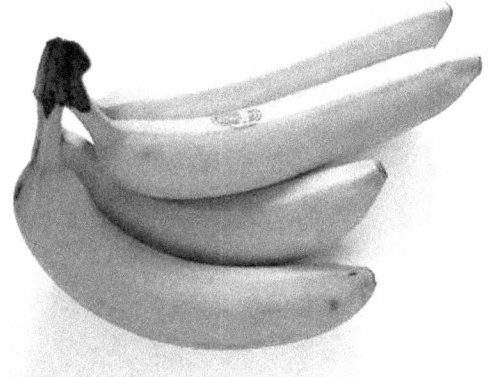

Image courtesy of 24oranges.nl

Bananas contain the highest
percentage of which vitamin?

   A. Pantothenic acid
   B. Vitamin B6
   C. Vitamin C

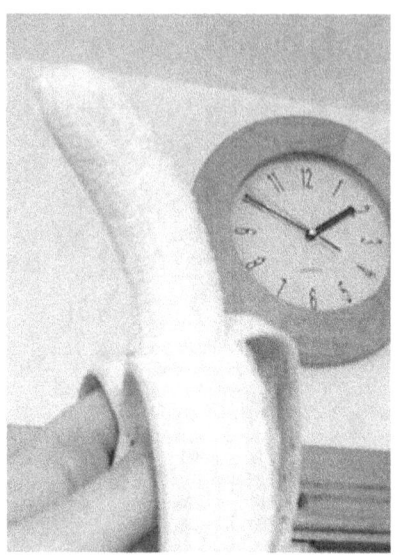

Image courtesy of Sean MacEntee

The answer is B. Vitamin B6

One medium banana provides almost 22% of the recommended daily intake (RDI) of vitamin B6. One medium banana provides about 6.5% RDI of pantothenic acid and less than 14% of the RDI of vitamin C.

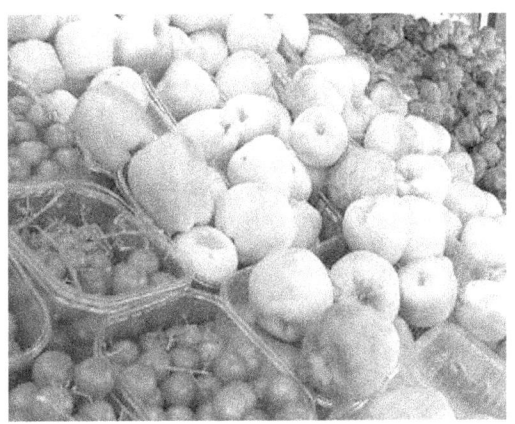

Image courtesy of miss pupik

Which fruit provides the most fiber?

A. Avocado
B. Pomegranates
C. Raisins

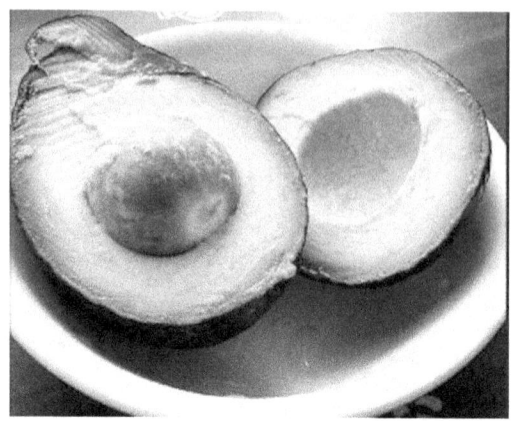

Image courtesy of You as a Machine

The answer is A. Avocado

One medium avocado provides about 13.5 grams of dietary fiber. One pomegranate provides about 11 grams and one small box of raisins provides less than 2 grams of fiber.

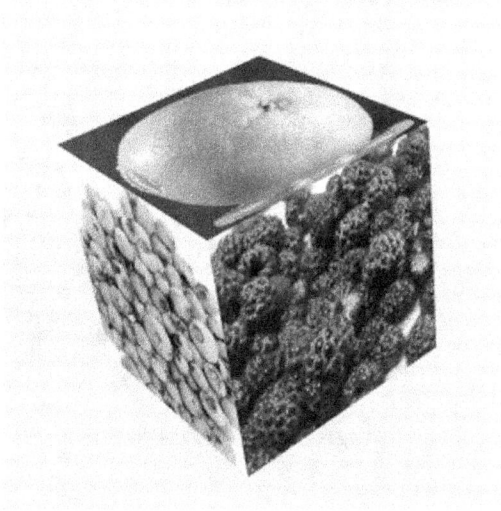

Images courtesy of wwwdotmetaphoricalplatypusdotcom (blueberries), Different Seasons Jewelry (boysenberries) and The Ewan (orange)

Of these three fruits, which one has the highest percentage of Folate?

A. Blueberries
B. Boysenberries
C. Oranges

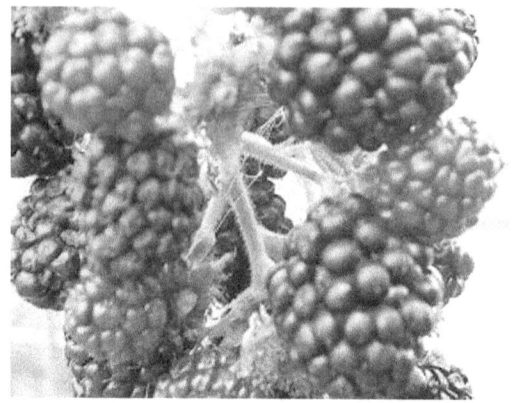

Image courtesy of Lnk.Si

The answer is B. Boysenberries

One cup of frozen boysenberries provides more than 20% of the recommended daily intake of Folate. One cup of blueberries provides just over 2% and one medium orange provides almost 10% of the RDI of Folate.

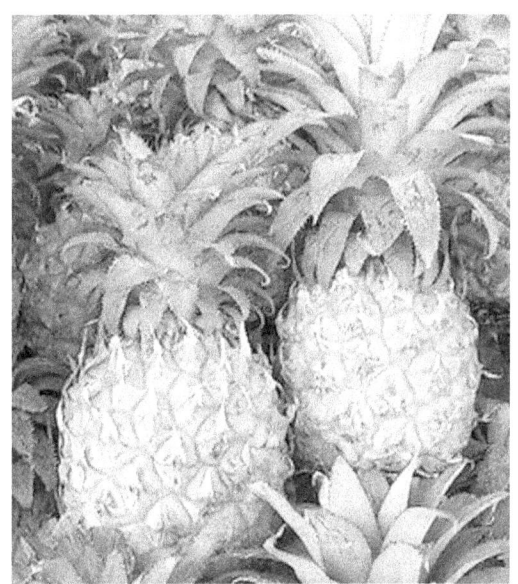

Image courtesy of Itinerant Tightwad

Pineapple contains the highest percentage of which vitamin?

A. Vitamin A
B. Vitamin B6
C. Vitamin C

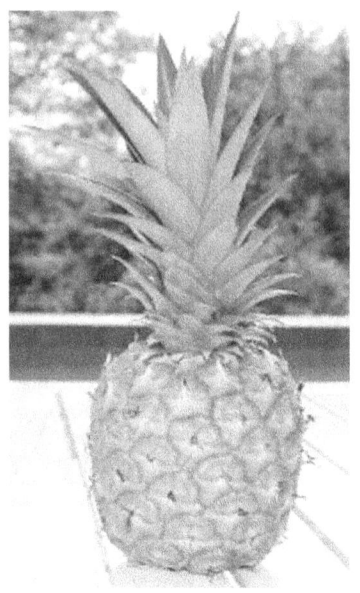

Image courtesy of public domain

The answer is C. Vitamin C

One cup of fresh pineapple chunks provides more than 100% of the recommended daily intake of vitamin C. It provides just less than 5% of the RDI of vitamin A and about 9% of the RDI of vitamin B6.

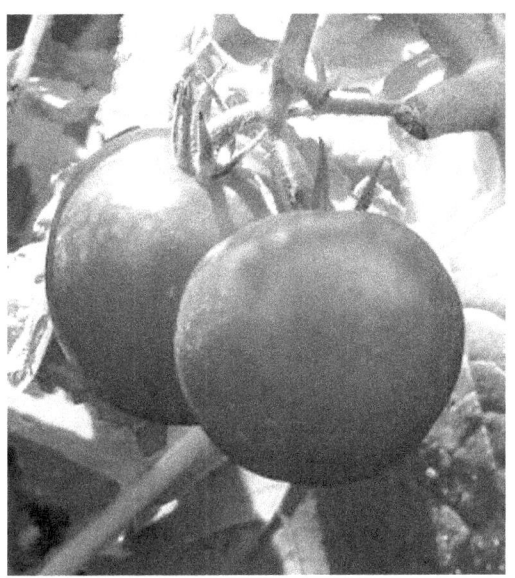

Image courtesy of Ajith chatie

Tomatoes contain the highest percentage of which vitamin?

A. Pantothenic acid
B. Vitamin A
C. Vitamin B6

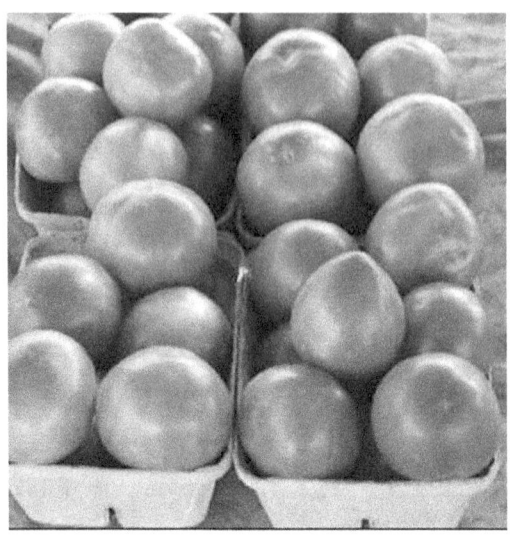

Image courtesy of La Grande Farmers Market

The answer is B. Vitamin A

One medium tomato provides about 51% of the recommended daily intake of vitamin A. It provides less than 2% of the RDI of pantothenic acid and about 5% of the RDI of vitamin B6.

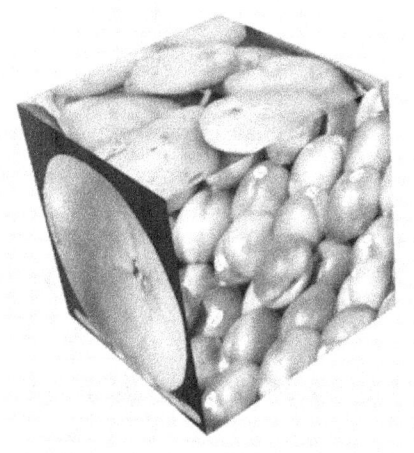

Images courtesy of TheGirlsNY
(nectarines), The Ewan (orange) and La
Grande Farmers Market (pears)

Of these three fruits, which one
has the highest percentage of
niacin?

    A. Nectarines
    B. Oranges
    C. Pears

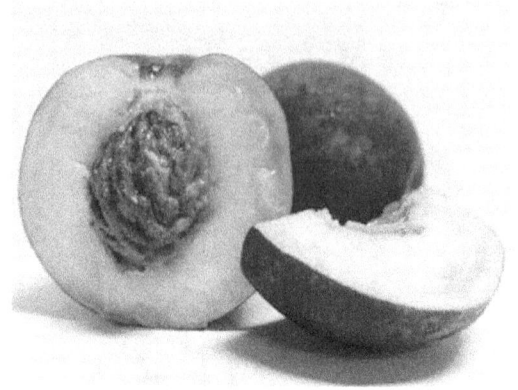

Image courtesy of travel oriented

The answer is A. Nectarines

One cup of sliced nectarines provides about 9% of the recommended daily intake of niacin. One medium orange only provides about 2% and one medium pear provides less than 2% of the RDI of niacin.

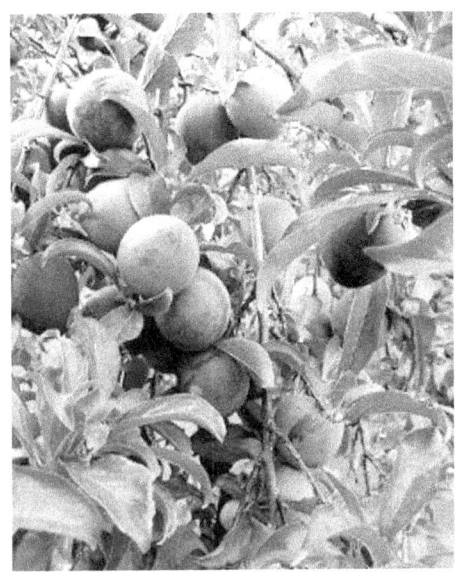

Image courtesy of cheekycrows3

Plums contain the highest percentage of which vitamin?

A. Vitamin A
B. Vitamin C
C. Vitamin K

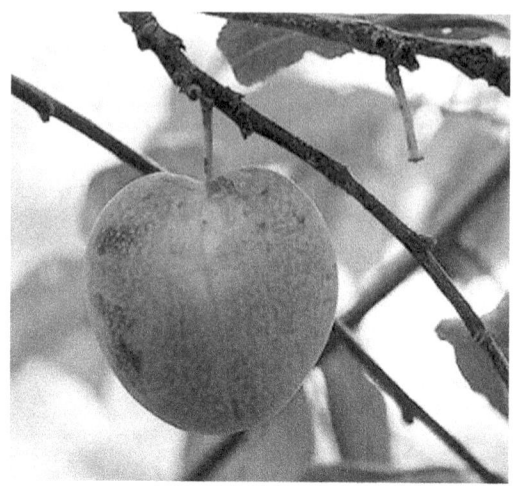

Image courtesy of cogdogblog

The answer is A. Vitamin A

One cup of sliced plums provides about 28% of the recommended daily intake of vitamin A. It provides almost 21% of the recommended daily intake of vitamin C and about 13% of the recommended daily intake of vitamin K.

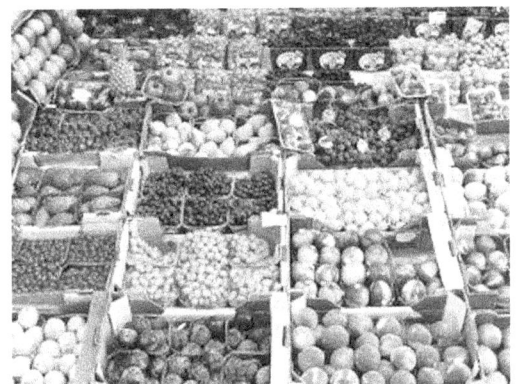

Image courtesy of Julien Lehuen

If you wanted the most of the mineral phosphorus possible, which of these three fruit is the best to eat?

A. Nectarines
B. Pomegranates
C. Raisins

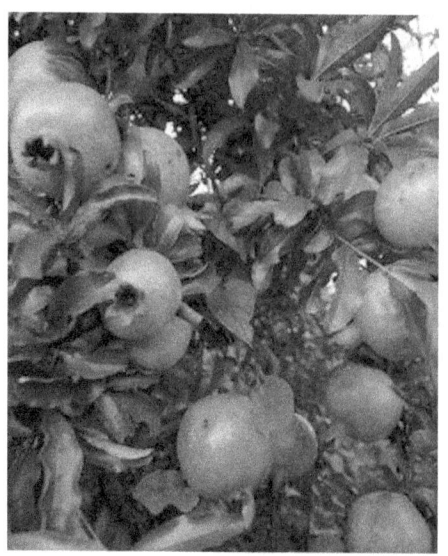

Image courtesy of matsuyuki

The answer is B. Pomegranates

One fresh pomegranate provides over 10% of the RDI of phosphorus. One cup of sliced nectarines provides just less than 4% and one small box of raisins provides just over 4% of the recommended daily intake of phosphorus.

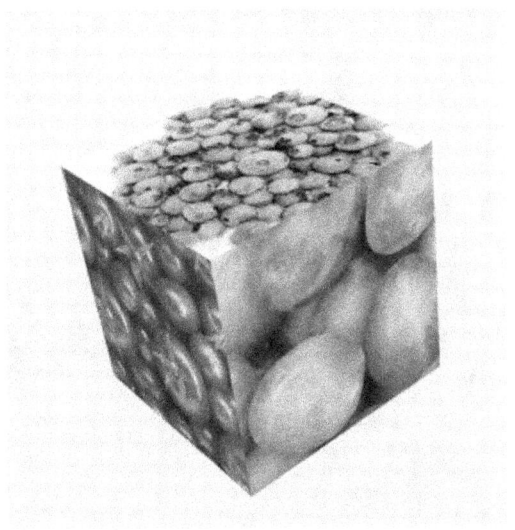

Images courtesy of metaphoricalplatypusdotcom (blueberries), ahisgett (plums) and The Ewan (tomatoes)

Of these three fruits, which one has the highest percentage of Vitamin E?

A. Blueberries
B. Plums
C. Tomatoes

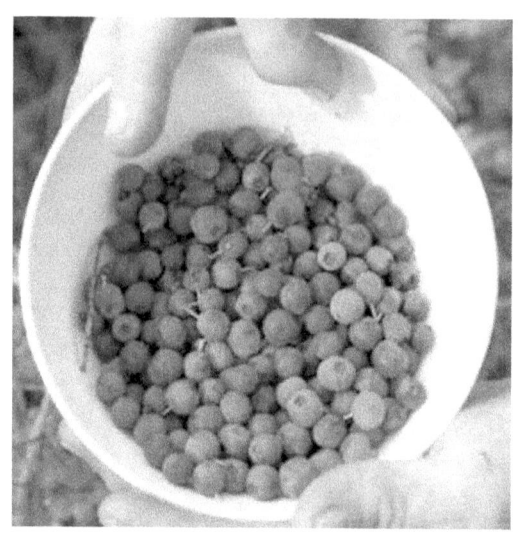

Image courtesy of public domain

The answer is A. Blueberries

One cup of blueberries provides almost 23% of the recommended daily intake of vitamin E. One cup of sliced plums provides the least vitamin E of these three fruits, at about 4%. One medium tomato provides about 6.5% of the RDI of vitamin E.

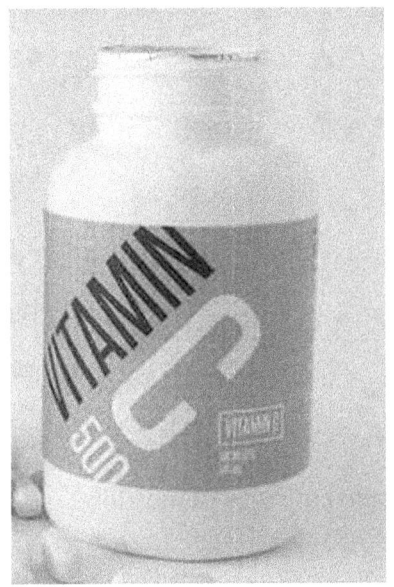

Image courtesy of colindunn

Which one of these three fruits gives you the highest percentage of Vitamin C?

   A. Lemons
   B. Oranges
   C. Tomatoes

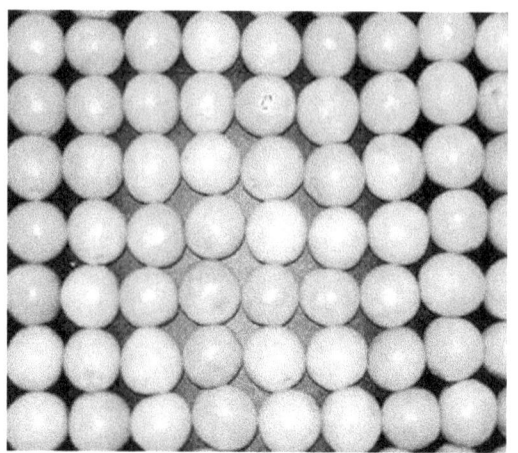

Image courtesy of mattieb

The answer is B. Oranges

One medium orange provides almost 93% of the recommended daily intake amount of vitamin C. One lemon (without peel) provides a lot of vitamin C at almost 60% of the RDI and one medium tomato provides a fair amount of vitamin C, about 21% of RDI.

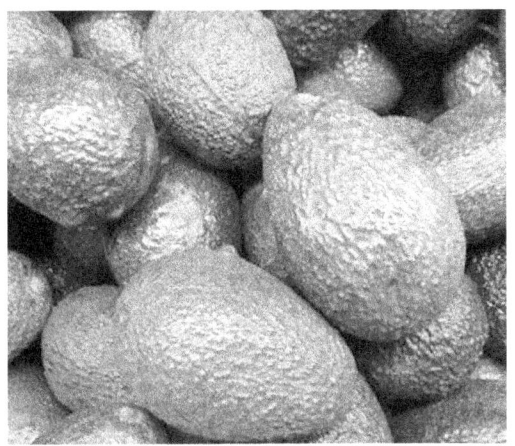

Image courtesy of ollesvensson

Avocados contain the highest percentage of which vitamin?

A. Pantothenic acid
B. Vitamin E
C. Vitamin K

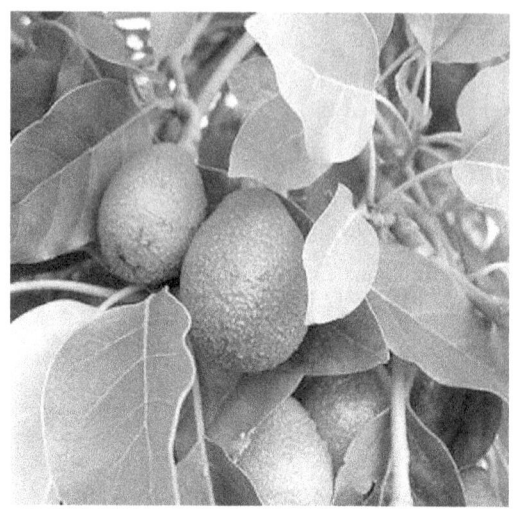

Image courtesy of avlxyz

The answer is C. Vitamin K

One medium avocado provides almost 53% of the recommended daily intake of vitamin K. One medium avocado provides over 46% of the recommended daily intake of pantothenic acid, and about 42% of the RDI of vitamin E.

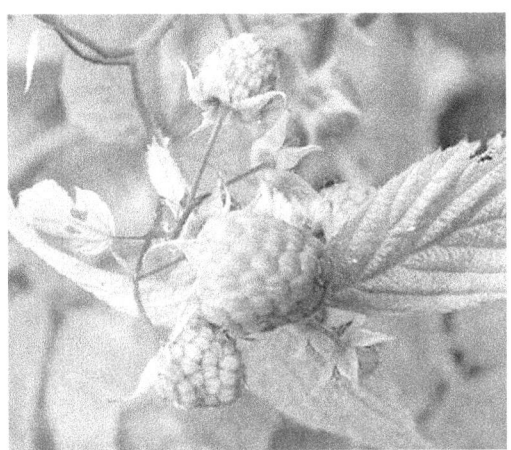

Image courtesy of MinivanNinja

Raspberries contain the highest percentage of which vitamin?

A. Folate
B. Niacin
C. Vitamin C

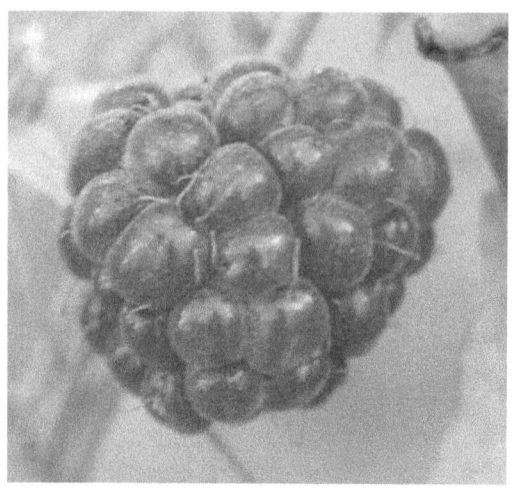

Image courtesy of public domain

The answer is C. Vitamin C

One cup of raspberries provides
almost 43% of the RDI of vitamin
C. One cup of raspberries
provides about 6.5% of the
recommended daily intake of
Folate, and about 4% of the
recommended daily intake of
niacin.

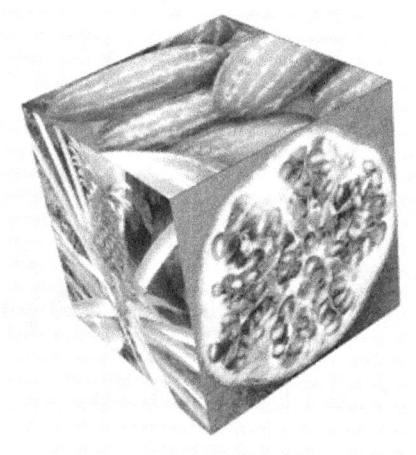

Images courtesy of derek7272
(pineapple), ahisgett (pomegranate),
and La Grande Farmers Market
(watermelon)

Of these three fruits, which one
has the highest percentage of
iron?

A. Pineapple
B. Pomegranate
    C. Watermelon

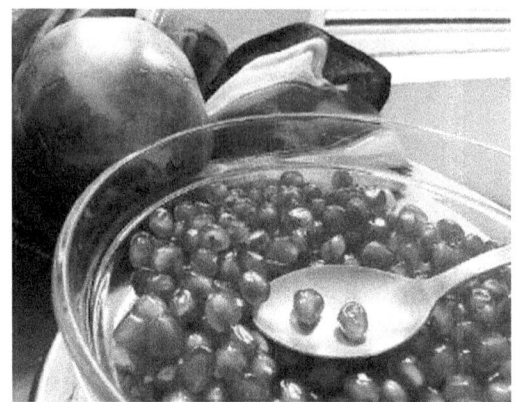

The answer is B. Pomegranate

One fresh pomegranate provides about 5.5% of the recommended daily intake of iron. One cup of fresh pineapple chunks provides about 3% and two cups of watermelon provide about 4.5% of the recommended daily intake of iron.

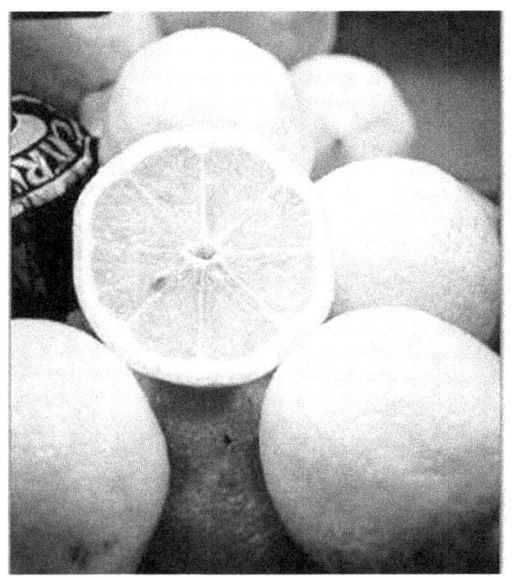

Image courtesy of Moyan Brenn

Lemons contain the highest percentage of which vitamin?

A. Niacin
B. Vitamin A
C. Vitamin C

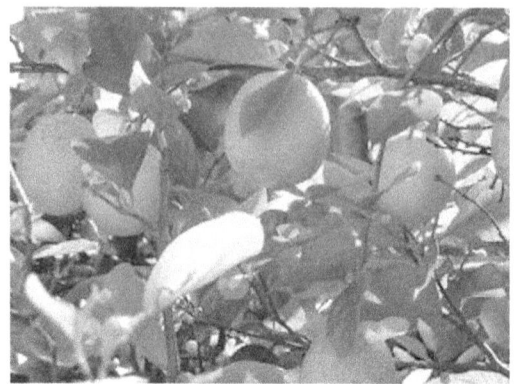

Image courtesy of Yellow Cat

The answer is C. Vitamin C

One lemon provides just over 59% of the recommended daily intake of vitamin C. One lemon without the peel provides less than 1% of the RDI of niacin and less than 1% of the RDI of vitamin A.

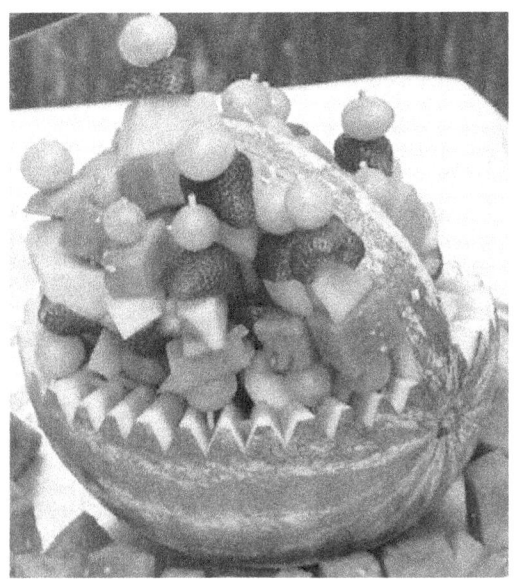

Image courtesy of burgundavia

If you wanted the most of the mineral iron possible, which fruit should you eat?

A. Boysenberries
B. Raisins
C. Watermelon

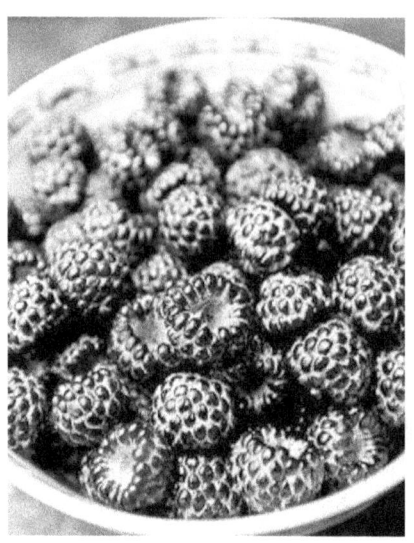

Image courtesy of sashafatcat

The answer is A. Boysenberries

One cup of frozen boysenberries provides the highest percentage at almost 7.5% of the recommended daily intake. One small box of raisins provides almost 5.5% and two cups of watermelon provide about 4.5% of the recommended daily intake of iron.

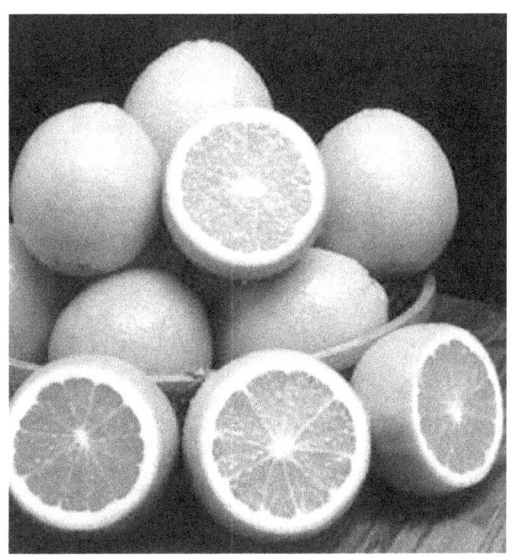

Image courtesy of public domain

Oranges contain the highest percentage of which vitamin?

A. Pantothenic acid
B. Vitamin C
C. Vitamin K

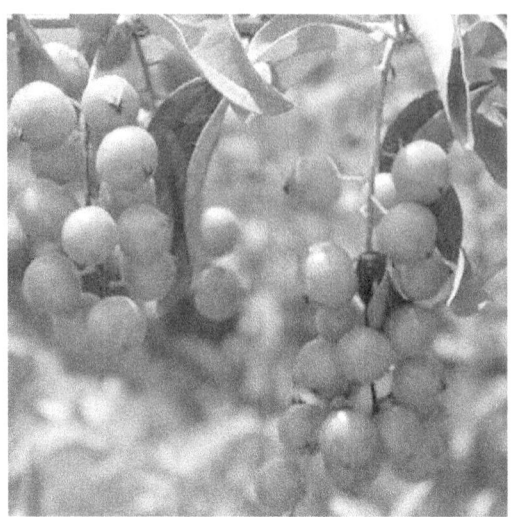

Image courtesy of Swami Stream

The answer is B. Vitamin C

One medium orange provides almost 93% of the RDI of vitamin C. It provides about 5.5% of the RDI of pantothenic acid. There is no vitamin K in oranges.

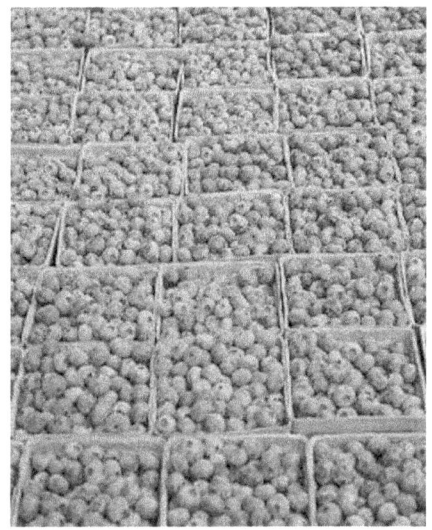

Image courtesy of prpmbd1050

Blueberries contain the highest percentage of which vitamin?

A. Vitamin C
B. Vitamin E
C. Vitamin K

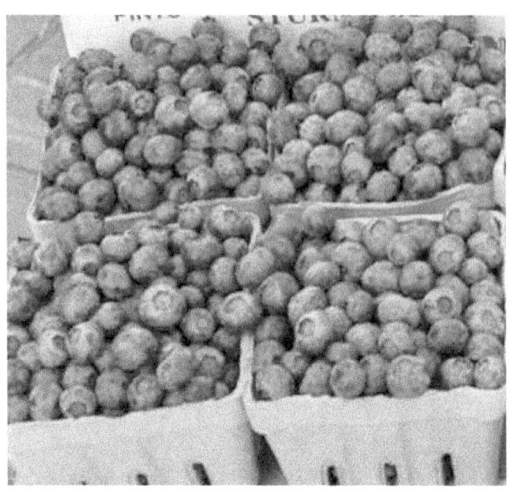

Image courtesy of La Grande Farmers Market

The answer is C. Vitamin K

One cup of blueberries provides almost 36% of the RDI of vitamin K. They provide about 19% of the recommended daily intake of vitamin C and almost 23% of the RDI of vitamin E.

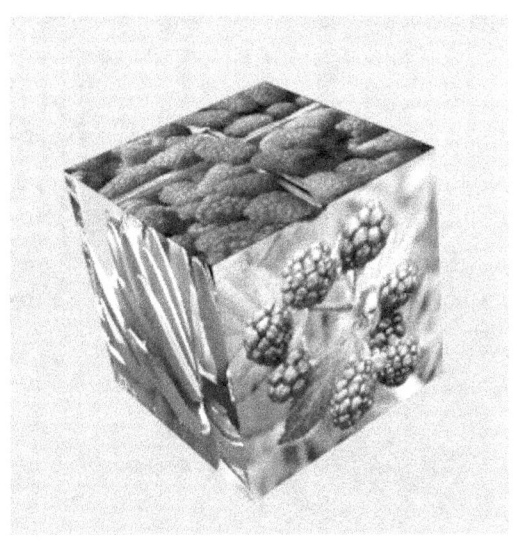

Images courtesy of librarianidol
(bananas), public domain
(blackberries), and La Grande Farmers
Market (raspberries)

Of these three fruits, which one
has the highest percentage of
potassium?

A. Bananas
B. Blackberries
C. Raspberries

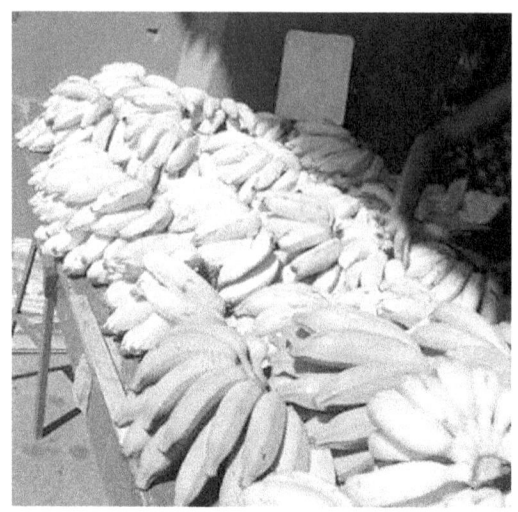

Image courtesy of jmarconi

The answer is A. Bananas

One medium banana provides about 12% of the recommended daily intake of potassium. One cup of blackberries provides about 6.5% and one cup of raspberries provides just over 5% of the RDI of potassium.

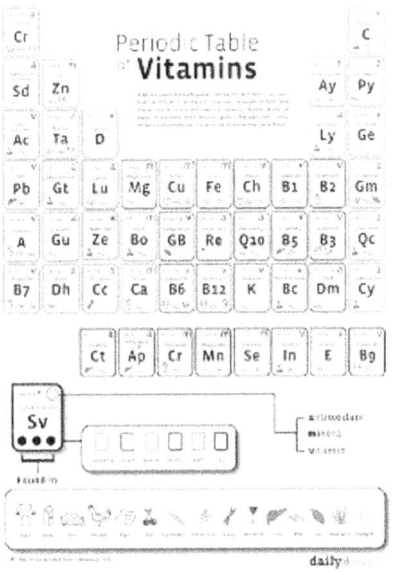

Image courtesy of stephanski

Which fruit provides the most
recommended daily Vitamin B1?

A. Grapes
B. Pomegranates
C. Watermelon

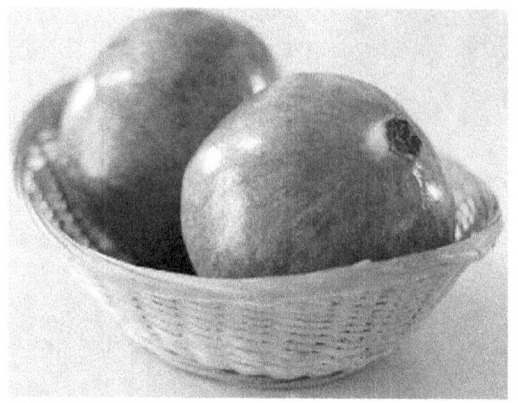

Image courtesy of melissa rae dale

The answer is B. Pomegranates

One pomegranate provides
about 13.5% of the
recommended daily intake of
vitamin B1. One cup of grapes
provides about 7.5% and two
cups of watermelon provide just
less than 7% of the RDI of
vitamin B1.

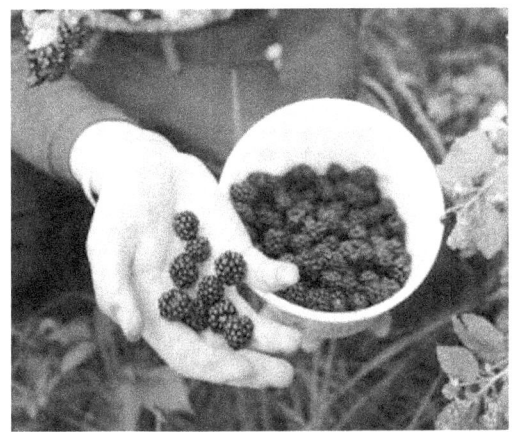

Image courtesy of public domain

Blackberries contain the highest percentage of which vitamin?

A. Vitamin C
B. Vitamin E
C. Vitamin K

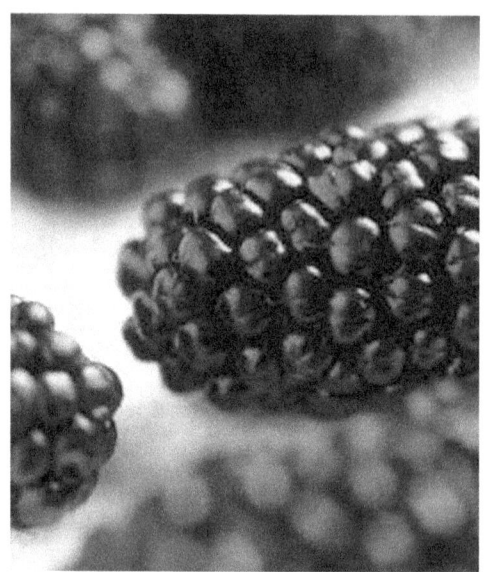

Image courtesy of public domain

The answer is A. Vitamin C

One cup of blackberries provides just over 40% of the recommended daily intake of vitamin C. They provide almost 17% of the recommended daily intake of vitamin E and almost 36% of the RDI of vitamin K.

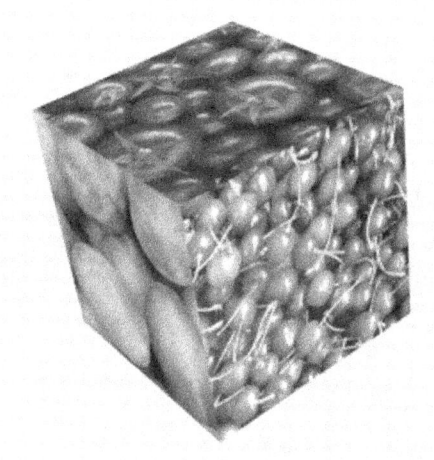

Images courtesy of La Grande Farmers Market (cherries), ahisgett (plums), and The Ewan (tomatoes)

Of these three fruits, which one has the highest percentage of zinc?

A. Cherries
B. Plums
C. Tomatoes

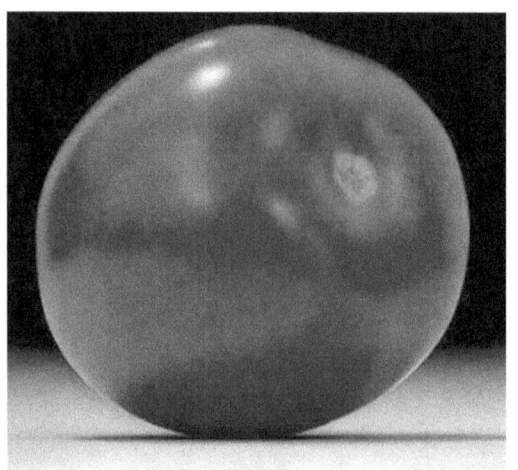

Image courtesy of Thomas Rousing

The answer is C. Tomatoes

While not very high in zinc at just less than 1.5% of the RDI, tomatoes provide the most zinc of this group. Watermelon, raspberries, pomegranates, avocados, and blackberries provide more zinc than tomatoes do.

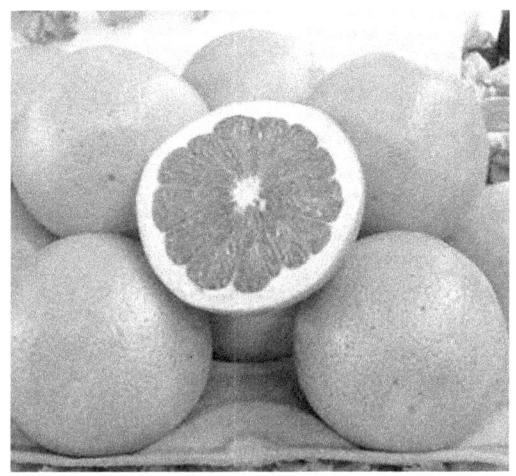

Image courtesy of Vic Lic

Grapefruit contain the highest percentage of which vitamin?

A. Vitamin A
B. Vitamin C
C. Vitamin E

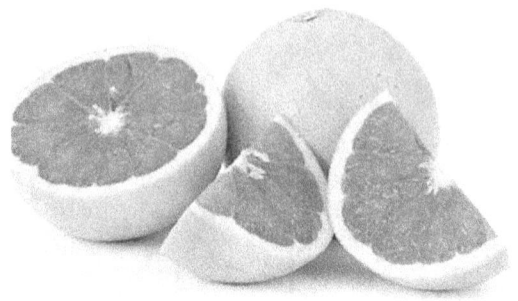

Image courtesy of dullhunk

The answer is A. Vitamin A

One cup of grapefruit barely provides a higher percentage of the RDI of vitamin A than vitamin C--almost 107% of the RDI of vitamin A compared to 105.5% of the RDI of vitamin C. It provides about 3% of the RDI of vitamin E.

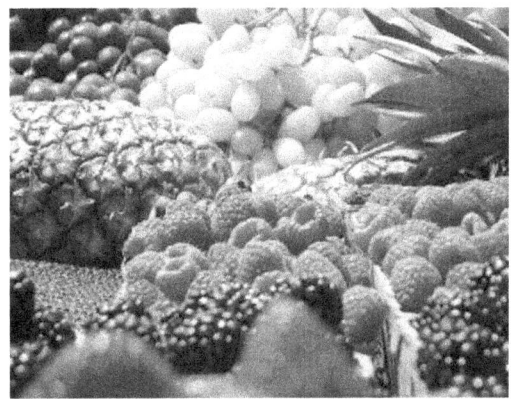

Image courtesy of plumandjello

If you wanted the most of the mineral manganese possible, which fruit should you eat?

A. Blackberries
B. Pineapple
C. Raspberries

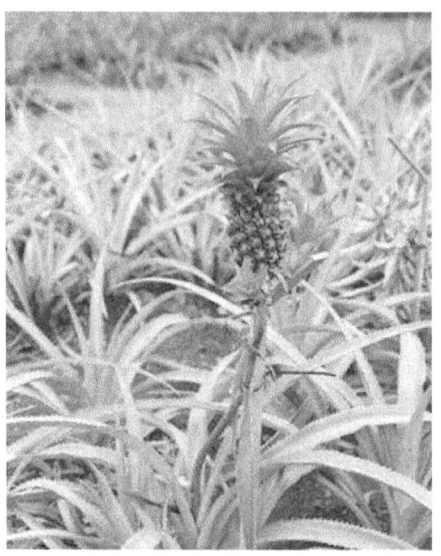

Image courtesy of cliff1066

The answer is B. Pineapple

Pineapples are great for manganese providing about 30% of the recommended daily intake. Blackberries are high in many vitamins and minerals, but manganese isn't one of them. One cup of raspberries provides

about 16% of the RDI of
manganese.

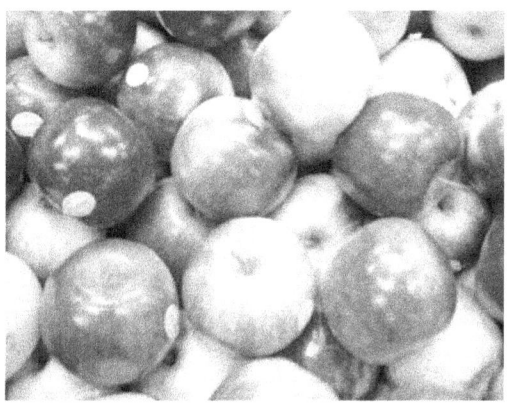

Image courtesy of public domain

Apples contain the highest
percentage of which vitamin?

- A. Vitamin A
- B. Vitamin C
- C. Vitamin K

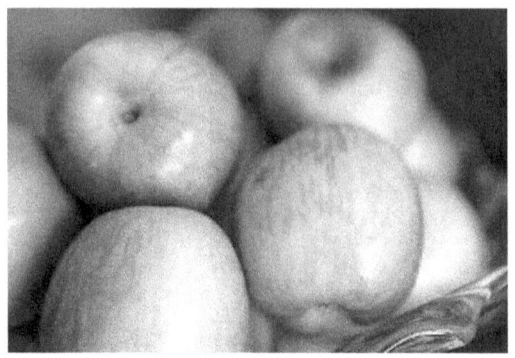

Image courtesy of planetc1

The answer is B. Vitamin C

One medium apple provides a little more than 11% of the recommended daily intake of vitamin C. It provides just less than 5% of the recommended daily intake of vitamin A and about 5% of the recommended daily intake of vitamin K.

Congratulations! You made it to the end!

The next time you shop for fruits you may have a better idea of the vitamins you are getting!

That was a lot of questions and you made it through all of them. Are you hungry for some fruit?

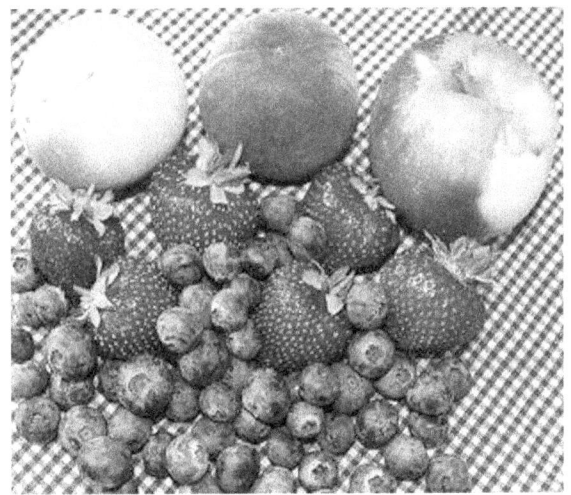

Image courtesy of the moment

Now you can impress or quiz or family and friends to see how much they know.

Look for more quiz books by Wyatt Michaels about presidents, states, dogs, horses, holidays, baseball, football, and more.

www.ingramcontent.com/pod-product-compliance
Lightning Source LLC
Chambersburg PA
CBHW070748290526
45795CB00002B/520